Kosiwa Ahonsou Dembele

Chronobiology and glycemic balance in type 1 diabetics

Kosiwa Ahonsou Dembele

Chronobiology and glycemic balance in type 1 diabetics

ScienciaScripts

Imprint

Cover image: www.ingimage.com

This book is a translation from the original published under ISBN 978-620-6-72072-0.

Publisher:
Sciencia Scripts
is a trademark of
Dodo Books Indian Ocean Ltd. and OmniScriptum S.R.L publishing group

120 High Road, East Finchley, London, N2 9ED, United Kingdom
Str. Armeneasca 28/1, office 1, Chisinau MD-2012, Republic of Moldova, Europe
Printed at: see last page
ISBN: 978-620-8-24234-3

DEDICATION

To my father and mother,

You are determined parents

THANKS

We thank the Lord Jesus Christ for his faithfulness and unfailing support.

Our gratitude to:

- M. DEMBELE Fangoura: your presence in my life helped me a lot in the realization of this work;
- My sisters and brothers, for your advice and prayers;
- My supervisors Dr. Demba DIEDHOU and Dr. Joseph NDONG for giving me their precious time and support throughout this thesis;
- To the Director of the Centre Marc Sankalé, Professor Saïd Norou Diop, for allowing me to carry out this work in the best possible conditions;
- All the staff of the Marc Sankalé Center, especially Faly SAMB and Binetou KEITA NDOYE;
- All type 1 diabetic patients who agreed to participate in this study;
- All the teachers of the Bio-Informatics course, especially Dr. Mouhamadou DIALLO, whom I thank warmly for all his support;
- The entire Groupe Biblique Universitaire de Dakar (G.B.U.D.) family, especially the BADIANE couple;
- To the COLE, GONDAMA and YAO families for their advice;
- To my brothers and sisters in Christ: Aimé MESSAN, David DUMENYA, Clémentine TITO and Patrick OUEDRAOGO.

SUMMARY

Chronobiology is the science of biological rhythms. It is constantly expanding its areas of application in the medical field, despite the fact that it has not yet been fully integrated into everyday practice. The aim of our study was to compare the results in terms of glycemic control between empirical and chronobiological control in type 1 diabetics at the Marc Sankalé Center (Dakar).

A prospective, cross-sectional study was conducted over a 6-month period. It included type 1 diabetic patients being monitored and educated in insulin therapy. A survey form was used to assess capillary blood glucose values, control times and insulin dose injected. The first step was for the patient to record his or her daily fasting capillary blood glucose at his or her usual blood glucose control times over a one-month period. Then, this same control was carried out according to a chronobiological rhythm, i.e. between 8 and 10 a.m. (the time interval when the acrophase of the glycemic rhythm occurs). The patient's HbA1c level was recorded at the end of each study phase. The data collected were entered and analyzed in Stata SE version 10 software to check whether there was a significant difference between blood glucose levels according to the two control methods. The test was significant when p-value<5%. The significance of the test influenced the parameters of the computerized insulin dose adjustment solution to be designed.

Nine (9) patients with a mean age of 27.2 years were included. Mean blood glucose and glycated hemoglobin levels were 1.71 g/l and 8.7% respectively in the conventional control group. For chronobiological control, mean blood glucose and HbA1c levels were 1.72 g/l and 9% respectively. There was no significant difference between blood glucose levels measured according to the biological clock and those measured according to the patient's usual clock (p-value>5%).

Our results reveal a lack of sufficient evidence to suggest that type 1 diabetic patients perform and interpret their glycemic controls according to the dynamic model proposed by chronobiology. This will require a larger comparative study.

Key words : Chronobiology - Glycemia - HbA1c levels

I. INTRODUCTION

Diabetes is a disease characterized by chronic hyperglycemia due to a deficiency in insulin production, resistance to insulin action, or a combination of both. Untreated hyperglycemia results in multiple complications that affect the whole body.

There are two main types of diabetes: type 1 and type 2. Type 1 diabetes most often manifests itself before adulthood. Its incidence peaks around 11-14 years of age. It is characterized by a complete absence of insulin production. Type 1 diabetics depend on daily injections of insulin to live. Type 2 diabetes manifests itself much later in life, generally around the age of 40. Today, however, it is increasingly being seen in younger people. Type 2 diabetes results from a combination of impaired insulin secretion and tissue insensitivity to insulin, known as insulin resistance. Type 2 diabetes, the most common form of diabetes, accounts for over 85% of cases .[1]

The incidence of diabetes worldwide, and particularly in sub-Saharan Africa, is rising at an alarming rate. This is contributing significantly to an increase in public health costs, as well as in diabetes-related loss of life.

The number of cases of diabetes rose from 30 million in 1985 to 135 million in 1995. This figure rose from 177 million in 2000 to 234 million in 2003[2] . In 2012, the number of diabetics worldwide was estimated at 371 million, according to the International Diabetes Federation (IDF). According to the latest estimates, the World Health Organization (WHO) suggests that 552 million people worldwide will have diabetes by 2030[3] . In sub-Saharan Africa, the number of diabetes cases was 12.1 million

---

[1] WHO Regional Office for Africa, Regional Director's Report, Diabetes prevention and control: a strategy for the WHO African Region, 2007

[2] *World Atlas 2003*, page 8/58.

[3] International Diabetes Federation, Global Diabetes Plan 2011-2021, [online], www.idf.org/sites/default/files/attachments/GDP_FR.pdf, accessed 12/02/14.

in 2010. If current trends continue, the number of diabetes cases in sub-Saharan Africa will reach 23.9 million by 2030[4] , an increase of 98%.

In Africa, like other non-communicable diseases, diabetes receives very little of the attention it deserves, despite its social, human and economic repercussions. Few countries have appropriate national programs and basic structures to combat this disease .[5]

Against this backdrop of massive growth in the prevalence of diabetes, diabetic care facilities such as the Centre Marc Sankalé, a benchmark facility in Senegal, are constantly involving all stakeholders (healthcare staff, social workers for therapeutic education, the State, donors, etc.) to better tackle this scourge.

However, *if you don't look in the right place, you won't find it*, says Dr. Jean-Michel Crabbé[6] . Indeed, modern medicine is failing to tackle the global diabetes epidemic because it looks to biology or genetics for the answers to lifestyle problems. We must never forget that it is biological rhythms that characterize life. "*Ignoring rhythms in biology, and particularly in medicine, can be compared to not washing your hands before surgery: the patient pays the price.* "Franz Halberg[7]

Chronobiology, which has been around since the 16th century, has been able to demonstrate the existence of endogenous physiological rhythms, as well as the pathologies that can be generated by disruption of these rhythms. Of course, not all human pathologies can be studied from this angle. But this approach can enrich our perception

---

[4] Observatoire Africain de la Sante, lutte contre le Diabète sucré, [online], www.aho.afro.who.int/profiles_information/index.php/...Diabetes.../fr, consulted on 12/02/14.

[5] WHO, Regional Office for Africa, op. cit. , p. 1.

[6] Jean-Michel Crabbé. SOS Diabète, [online], www.sitemed.fr/diabète, accessed 03/03/13.

[7] Halberg, Franz. Solving some generally applicable chronobiological puzzles. *Bulletin du groupe d'étude des rythmes biologiques*, 1989, no. 1, pp. 36-52.

and understanding of diseases such as diabetes. For example, knowledge of the ultradian rhythms of diabetics enables dynamic analysis of patients' blood sugar levels, and provides a degree of therapeutic anticipation that is beneficial to the management of these patients.

In view of the rhythmic functioning of organs, it is therefore interesting to study their reactions to drug administration. In the management of type 1 diabetics, what role does the time factor play in glycemic control? Is there a difference between the results of blood glucose checks performed according to patients' usual schedules and those of blood glucose checks performed according to the biological clock? Is chronobiological control advantageous for patients' glycemic control? What computerized solution can be proposed to type 1 diabetic patients for better adaptation of their insulin dose?

II. BACKGROUND AND RATIONALE

Diabetes is now presented as a multifactorial disease, combining environmental triggers, predisposing genetic factors and an immune response. In 2006, the WHO defined type 1 diabetes as a disease characterized by insufficient insulin secretion, rapidly fatal without daily administration of insulin . [8]

Indeed, the progressive death of islet β-cells is responsible for insulin deficiency and a loss of homeostatic blood glucose balance. Thus, Grimaldi was able to assert that *type 1 diabetes is due to autoimmune destruction of insulin-producing β-cells. This process occurs in a favorable genetic background, following environmental triggers .*[9]

Since the 1920s, substitute treatment with daily doses of insulin has enabled diabetics to lead almost normal lives. Today, hand-held blood glucose meters and biogenetic insulins such as analogues significantly improve these treatments, and new methods are currently being evaluated or marketed.

This therapeutic model has amply demonstrated its usefulness: for over eighty (80) years, it has saved diabetics from certain death and enabled them to live almost normally. It can also be used to treat diabetic comas and other complications of diabetes.

Many arguments, especially those of chronobiologists, prove that this definition of type 1 diabetes, inherited from the 19th century, remains highly inadequate and should be abandoned. However, this classic theory, based on the principle of glycemic homeostasis, is the one taught and present in all endocrinology textbooks.

---

[8] WHO. Diabetes: Fact Sheet n°312, September 2006.

[6] Grimaldi A. Diabétologie. Questions d'internat 1999 - 2000. Pierre and Marie Curie Faculty of Medicine. University of Paris VI.

Indeed, according to Claude Bernard[10] and his students, the environment of organisms is constant (homeostasis) and any change or disturbance will be corrected by a counter-reaction (retrocontrol, feedback), enabling the organism to return to the previous level. This gave rise to the notion of the "biological constant": levels of glucose, cholesterol, hormones, enzymes and red blood cells would be constant. Any variation in their levels would be due to stress, dietary intake or a pathological condition: a counter-reaction by the organism would normally bring it back to the level preceding the "disturbance".

Reinberg's work since 1970 has shown that this is not the case! All these "biological constants" vary according to cycles. The amplitude of these cycles can span a fraction of a second, a day, a year or a lifetime. It is therefore more correct to speak of "physiological variables" rather than biological constants. Depending on the time of day or age, the results of blood or biological analyses can become incomparable. This is why, if you want to be able to interpret these tests correctly, they should always be carried out at the same time.

Chronobiology refers to the enzymatic and hormonal secretions of the human organism, whose variations or appearances are inescapably regulated by hourly stimuli of activity, light or night or sleep, cold or heat, hunger or satiety.

Scientists have thus been able to pinpoint certain fundamental human stimuli: sunrise, sunset, fatigue, thirst, hunger and, more recently, stimuli linked to the start or end of activity of the various digestive organs. The mechanisms governing homeostasis are far from the only ones involved in metabolic equilibrium. All living organisms, however complex, have biological rhythms.

The internal rhythms that animate animal and plant species have been known and studied since antiquity. According to Dr. Jean-Michel Crabbé, *the ancients noticed the*

---

[10] Famous 19th-century French physiologist

differences between nocturnal and diurnal species. They studied the cycles of reproduction, activity and rest, migration and hibernation of many animal species[11] . Chronobiology was born of this concern to improve the best conditions for living organisms in their biotope: first among botanists, then among zoologists.

It is therefore the science of the rhythmic organization of living beings. It has recently made considerable progress in extending its application to the medical field. Chronobiology *concerns all fundamental disciplines such as cell biology and physiology, as well as the various medical specialties* .[12]

Chronobiology studies bodily rhythms by taking time into account in the physiological functioning of the organism. In the field of medicine, chronobiology covers a wide field, and its clinical implications are beginning to permeate practices such as *the performance of biological assays, particularly hormonal assays, at a precise time of day to ensure reliable results. This is because fluctuations can sometimes vary by as much as 200% depending on the time of day*[13] , notes Eric Marsaudon.

In diabetology, chronobiology provides a better understanding of the fluctuations in blood sugar levels that mark patients' equilibrium, and allows us to understand the dynamics of human physiology and pathologies.

Chronobiological studies have been carried out to determine the rhythmicity of insulin secretion[14] : fast and slow oscillations, as well as glycemic oscillations[15] . This made it possible, on the one hand, to study endogenous dysfunctions of insulin secretion

---

[11] Jean Michel Crabbé, De la biologie à la chronobiologie, [online], www.sitemed.fr, consulted on 30/08/12.

[12] Jean-Michel Crabbé, Médecine et chronobiologie, I. les origines de la chronobiologie. L'échec de la médecine occidentale: l'idéologie médicale en question, *Ellébore* ,2003 :167-170.

[13] Eric Marsaudon, La chronobiologie, une conception dynamique du fonctionnement corporel, *Presses de Sciences Po | Les Tribunes de la santé* 2006/4 - no 13 ; 39-44 ISSN 1765-8888.

[14] Simon C. Brandenberger G., La pulsabilité de l'insulinosécrétion, *Rev Prat*(Paris) 1994; 44, 6: 791-94.

[15] Middeke M. Schrader J., Nocturmi blood pressure in normotensive subjects and those with white cont. primary and secondary hypertension, *BMJ* 1994; 308:630-632.

in type 2 diabetic patients, and the sensitivity of peripheral receptors. But also to assess the role of counter-regulatory hormones in type 1 diabetics, on the other hand[16] . These pathophysiological aspects of type 1 diabetes led G.B. Bolli[17] to consider an alternative pharmacokinetic form of insulin for better control of morning hyperglycemia.

While the notion of homeostasis seems to be firmly anchored in medical procedures, the medical world is surprisingly open to the dynamic interpretation of biological data. Indeed, it has been shown that *taking time into account in patient monitoring was already a notion intuitively perceived by diabetologists, who have long noted unexplained glycemic fluctuations in their patients, be they nycthemeral, monthly or annual*[18] .

Chronobiologists have had the merit of devising mathematical models such as the "cosinor" model, and others derived from[19] spectral analysis, to carry out rhythmic readings of the various organic functions.

---

[16] Jean Michel Crabbé, De la biologie à la chronobiologie, op. cit. , p. 13.

[17] Bolli G.B., Circadian rhythms of insulin sensitivity and its role in the treatment of diabetes mellitus. In Biological cloks. Mechanisms and applications. Amsterdam *Elsevier Science* 1998: 405-409

[18] Eric Marsaudon, Chronobiologie et diabète. *Rev La semaine des Hôpitaux de Paris* ,1998 ; 74 : 1148-1154.

[19] Nelson W, Tong YL, Lee J-K, Halberg F. Methods for cosinor rhythmometry. Chronobiologia, 1979;6:305-23.
See also:
Bourdon L, Buguet A, Cucherat M, Radomski MW. Use of a spreadsheet program for circadian analysis of biological/physiological data. Aviat Space Environ Med, 1995; 66: 787-91.

Sokolove PG, Bushell WN. The chi square periodogram: its utility for analysis of circadian rhythms. *J Theor Biol*, 1978; 8: 131-60.

We used the rhythmicity of the pancreas, in particular glycemic oscillations, as the basis for a comparative study of the results of conventional and chronobiological blood glucose monitoring in nine (09) type 1 diabetic patients. The comparative study was also carried out on the results of patients' glycated hemoglobin (HbA1c) assays at the end of each control method to assess their glycemic control.

In fact, independently of food intake, blood glucose levels follow a circadian rhythm, with acrophase around 10 a.m. and batiphase around 4 p.m.[20] . The timing of blood glucose control is therefore fundamental to interpretation.

The notion of biological rhythmicity or chronobiology seems to be ignored in African medical circles. It is therefore important to carry out a comparative study on the timing of blood glucose monitoring. This is because glycemic controls have a major influence on insulin dose adaptation in type 1 diabetics.

Treatment of type 1 diabetes must enable young diabetics to lead lives as competitive as those of non-diabetics. *Since the early 80s, self-monitoring of blood glucose has been introduced in the treatment of insulin-dependent diabetics*[21] *. The possibility for patients to perform their own capillary blood glucose tests is one of the most important technical advances in insulin-dependent* diabetes[22] . Self-monitoring of blood glucose levels is therefore an essential part of diabetes management.

For better follow-up, patients should record the results of their blood and/or urine tests in a diary, which should be presented to the nursing staff for evaluation. These results will be useful for adjusting diet and insulin dosage, and for defining new treatment objectives.

---

[20] Jean-Michel Crabbé, Médecine et chronobiologie, op. cit. , p. 7.

[21] S. Halimi. Contributions of self-monitoring of blood glucose in the management of insulin-dependent (IDDM) and non-insulin-dependent (NIDDM) diabetics. *Diabetes & Metabolism* 1998, 24, 35-41.

[22] Tattersall R. Homme glucose monitoring. *Diabetologia,* 1979, 16: 71-74

Patients undergoing insulin therapy at the Centre Marc Sankalé are accustomed to recording their glycemic and ketone control in a thirty-two (32) page notebook. With the help of the nursing staff, they can easily adapt the insulin dose they need to inject daily.

Thanks to the STATA software's comparison tests, this study aims to :

- Verify whether there is a significant difference between the results of conventional control and those of chronobiological blood glucose control.

- Appreciate the contribution of computer science to the scientific resolution of biological problems. An algorithm implemented in Java language will be proposed to type 1 diabetics to better adapt their insulin dose.

The subject will therefore be approached from a statistical and IT angle.

III. MATERIALS AND METHODS

1. Scope and type of study

It was a prospective, descriptive study conducted from January 01 to June 12, 2013. The study was conducted at the Clinique Médicale II of the Centre Hospitalier Abass Ndao in Dakar. It comprises 2 departments, namely the Marc Sankalé Diabetes Center and the Internal Medicine Service.

The Marc Sankalé Diabetes Center is the national reference center for the management of endocrine and metabolic pathologies. This care takes the form of outpatient consultations by appointment, and emergency consultations for acute complications of diabetes and diabetic foot lesions. The center houses a podiatry room specially equipped for the monitoring and prevention of at-risk feet, and a department for therapeutic education.

Hospitalisation takes place in the internal medicine department run by the same medical team. This department caters for all pathologies requiring internal medical care, but diabetics predominate. The 36-bed department is divided into two wings, A and B, for female and male patients respectively.

The Medical Clinic II of the Abass Ndao Hospital Center is a university hospital department with medical and paramedical staff. It is under the responsibility of a professor in charge of the department, assisted by two associate professors and two assistants. In addition to medical care, these staff are also involved in university teaching and research. The rest of the staff is made up of seven (7) interns and, of course, the paramedical staff of twenty-seven (27) nurses, including two ward supervisors.

Two social workers are responsible for therapeutic patient education. Discussions take the form of a debate, preceded by a presentation on the therapeutic and preventive aspects of diabetes.

2. STUDY POPULATION

The study population consisted of type 1 diabetic patients of all ages and genders, known and followed at the Marc Sankalé Center.

3. SAMPLING AND INCLUSION CRITERIA

It consisted in selecting, by simple random sampling, a sample of patients from among type 1 diabetics who met the inclusion criteria and had agreed to take part in the study following free and informed consent. Our study included type 1 diabetic patients who were already familiar with and educated about the various aspects of diabetes mellitus management. Patients should have a minimum knowledge of diabetes and self-monitoring practices. They must also meet the following profile:

- Own and operate an Accu-Chek ACTIVE meter;
- To be regularly monitored by the Marc Sankalé Center;
- Being "physically" healthy.

Patients who did not meet the above criteria and those who did not consent to participate in the survey were not included.

4. DATA COLLECTION PROCEDURE

Over a total period of sixty (60) days, each patient had to perform capillary fasting blood glucose tests every morning. Monthly glycated hemoglobin measurements were also taken. These results were recorded on a survey form[23] supplied by the investigator. The data collected on this form included the patient's age and sex, date and time of blood glucose control, morning capillary blood glucose values, insulin dose injected and monthly HbA1c results.

---

[23] See appendix

In the first phase, diabetic patients were asked to fill in survey forms according to their usual blood glucose control times over the course of a month. They were asked to mention the times of control, the morning fasting blood glucose results, and the doses of insulin injected. At the end of the study period, they measured glycated hemoglobin. This is the classic control technique.

In a second phase, the same diabetics repeated the study over a one-month period. This time, an hourly interval was set for blood glucose control. Since the acrophase of the glycemic rhythm occurred between 8 and 10 a.m., these diabetics had to do their control within this time interval. The results of their glycated hemoglobin measurements were recorded again at the end of this second stage of the study. This technique is known as chronobiological control.

5. CAPILLARY BLOOD GLUCOSE TEST METHOD

The Accu-Chek Active meter is designed for quantitative blood glucose determination using fresh capillary blood and test strips.

The Accu-Chek Active meter uses an electrochemical method: the blood on the test strip comes into contact with an enzyme (glucose oxidase) and the chemical reaction produces an oxidation, with the production of electrons, and therefore an electric current, detected by the device and proportional to the amount of glucose. To measure blood glucose levels, proceed as follows:

- Wash or disinfect hands and dry.
- Place the strip in the reader.
- prick your finger with the finger pricker to obtain a drop of blood
- Apply the drop to the strip.

The result, expressed in mg/dl, appears on the meter's display in a few seconds. The lancet and strip are disposed of in accordance with the relevant instructions.

Figures 1 and 2 show a representative illustration of an Accu-Chek Active finger-stick blood glucose monitoring device.

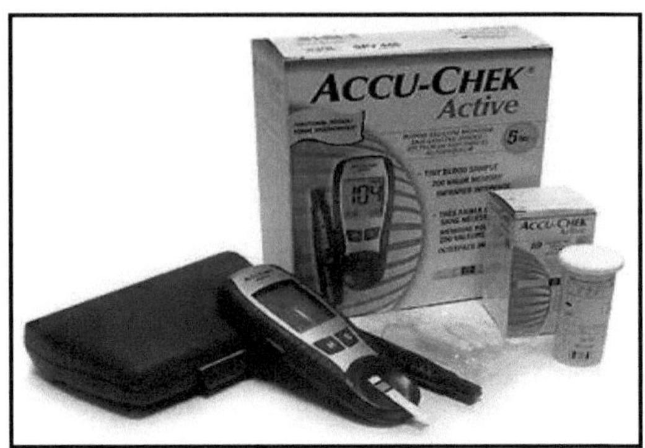

Figure 1 Glycometer with spike and test strip

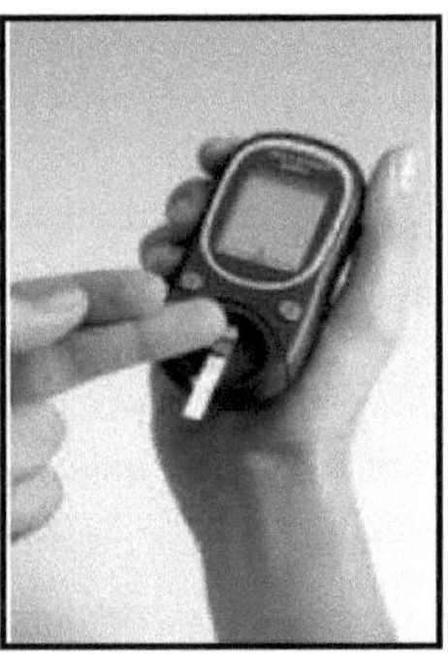

Figure 2Glycometer for blood glucose monitoring

6. GLYCATED HEMOGLOBIN MEASUREMENT METHOD

This is done by measuring a specific component of red blood cells, the hemoglobin A1c molecules. Through a non-enzymatic glycation process, glucose binds to A1c molecules as they circulate in the bloodstream. High-performance liquid chromatography (HPLC) is used to measure HbA1c. Figure 3 shows a machine used to determine glycated hemoglobin.

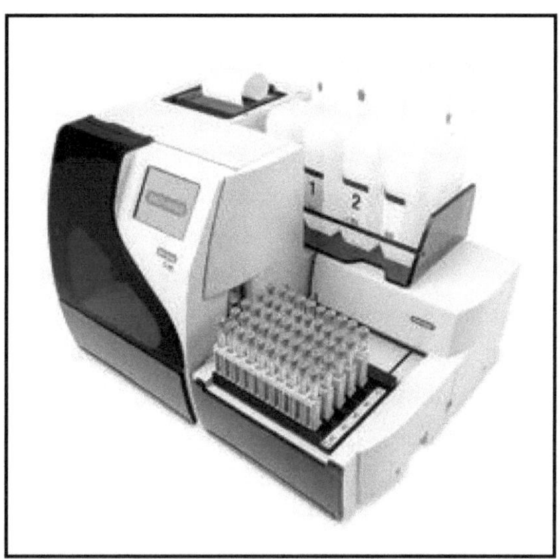

Figure 3 D-10 hemoglobin analyzer™ Rack Loader

The D-10™ hemoglobin analyzer from Bio-Rad Laboratories consists of two (2) modules: a chromatographic module and a sample processing module. The D-10™ HbA1c test is a fully automated method that delivers HbA1c assay results in 3 minutes. Primary tube sampling eliminates sample preparation steps, lightening the user's workload. The D-10™ delivers accurate and reliable results.

The sample to be analyzed is pushed by a liquid (called the mobile phase) through a column filled with a fine-grain stationary phase[24] . The flow rate of the mobile phase is high, which increases the pressure in the system. This high flow rate reduces the time required to separate the components along the stationary phase. The fine particle size of the stationary phase also enhances component separation. Indeed, for the same volume of stationary phase, the exchange surface area increases if the "grains" that make it up are

[24] The "grains" are very small in size

smaller in diameter. The resulting peaks are narrower, so resolution is improved[25] , and the detection threshold is also lower[26] . The combination of these attributes - speed and high resolution - leads to the name "high performance".

For each sample analyzed, the D-10™ prints a report containing the following information: sample type (calibrant, control, patient), patient identification, injection identification (serial number, rack number, sample position on the rack), areas and retention times of the various peaks identified, HbA1c level and chromatogram. For normal blood, six fractions are identified and quantified: HbA1a, HbA1b, HbF, labile HbA1c identified as "LA1c" on the report, HbA1c, HbAo (in order of elution). The area of the HbA1c peak is calculated using a modified Gaussian exponential function algorithm[27] which subtracts labile HbA1c and carbamylated Hb (eluted in the "LA1c" peak). The peak transformed by the algorithm is shown shaded on the chromatogram (fig.4).

---

[25] The peaks are well separated, so they are clearly distinguishable.

[26] Narrow, high peaks are easier to isolate from background noise than wide, low peaks

[27] Foley JP, Dorsey JG. A review of the exponentially modified gaussian (EMG) function: evaluation and subsequent calculation of universal data. J Chromatogr Sci 1984; 22: 40-6.

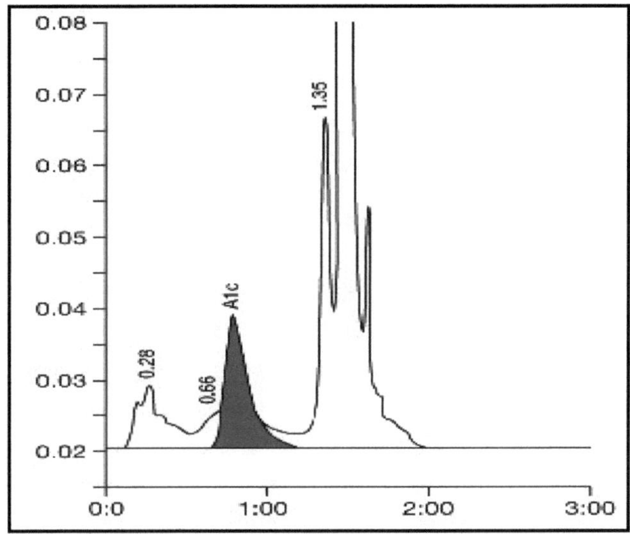

Figure 4Example of a chromatogram

7. OPERATIONAL DEFINITION OF VARIABLES

- Blood sugar levels

This is the concentration of glucose in the blood. It is said to be fasting for a blood glucose level measured in the morning after fasting for 8 to 12 hours. The result is normal if it is between 70 and 100 mg/dl for preprandial blood glucose, or below 160 mg/dl for postprandial blood glucose. Hypoglycemia occurs when the blood glucose result is below 70 mg/dl. Hyperglycemia occurs when the result is above 110 mg/dl for preprandial blood glucose, or above 160 mg/dl for postprandial blood glucose.

- HbA1c levels

Glycated hemoglobin or HbA1c reflects the average blood glucose level over a period of 2 to 3 months.

Normal values: 4.8 to 6%.

Glycemic balance < 7%.

8. Data capture and analysis

The comparative study focused on fasting capillary blood glucose and glycated hemoglobin results from patients in these two control phases. *Treatment efficacy was judged by the repeated glycated hemoglobin levels that should be maintained under 7%*[28]

.

First, the independent variables (or factors) of the study were isolated: the patient variable **p** (n=9), and the control variable **c**, which had two modalities ($\mathbf{c_1}$: classical control; $\mathbf{c_2}$: chronobiological control). The dependent variable was blood glucose value (in g/l) or Hb1Ac level (in %). Since blood glucose and HbA1c measurements were repeated on each patient during both control phases, a matched-group design was used. Data were summarized in the form of a[29] data table, exportable from Microsoft Excel to STATA.

- **Microsoft Excel**

Microsoft Excel is an office spreadsheet program for data analysis. The software's grouped histograms can already be used to visualize comparisons.

- **STATA SE**

Stata is a statistical and econometric software package that works with command lines typed in by the user. It is particularly used by the scientific community for research in medicine, biology and economics. Stata SE is a professional version with the ability to calculate large datasets.

---

[28] H. Dorchy, Insulin choice and dose adaptation in diabetic children and adolescents: personal experience, *Rev Méd Brux* 2000; 1 :19-27.

[29] See table 3, p.46.

Stata SE version 10 was used to calculate the test statistic for comparison of blood glucose or HbA1c averages from the two data sets[30] . First, we chose the statistical test that would verify the acceptability of the research hypothesis. The research hypothesis stated that there was no significant difference between the two types of blood glucose and HbA1c control. We then carried out a statistical test, setting out the hypotheses for comparison.

The assumptions for comparing blood glucose averages were[31] :

$$H_0 : m_1 = m_2$$

$$H_1 : m_1 > m_2$$

The assumptions for comparing mean HbA1c levels were[32] :

$$H_0 : m'_1 = m'_2$$

$$H_1 : m'_1 > m'_2$$

The choice of statistical test to accept or reject these various null hypotheses[33] required prior verification of the normality of the distribution of blood glucose levels and HbA1c levels obtained. Thus, the parametric Student's t test will be used in the case of a Gaussian distribution, and the non-parametric Wilcoxon test in the case of a non-Gaussian distribution.

---

[30] Classic control and chronobiological control

[31] H_1 : null hypothesis; H_2 : alternative hypothesis;

m_1 : average of blood glucose levels from classic control m ; 2 : average of blood glucose levels from chronobiological control.

[32] m'_1 : average HbA1c levels from classical control ; m'_2 : average HbA1c levels from chronobiological control.

[33] The test is significant when p<5%.

The *Student's t test* for comparing two means (of blood glucose or HbA1c levels) is a parametric test whose formula contains 4 estimators (ml, m2, s1, s2)[34] and whose probability distribution of the statistic under H_0 follows a Student's law. The STATA command used to perform this test is: *ttest varname1 = = varname2.*

The *Wilcoxon test* is an alternative to *Student's t-test.* Here, the differences between matched values are calculated and then ranked in ascending order of absolute values, omitting zero differences. Each non-zero difference is assigned its rank in the ranking. The Stata command for a Wilcoxon signed-rank test is: *signtest varname1 = varname2*

Since self-monitoring of blood glucose has an influence on the dose of insulin that the patient must inject, a computerized solution for adapting the insulin dose should be proposed. The parameters of the IT platform for insulin dose adaptation depended on the acceptability or otherwise of the research hypothesis. Thus, these parameters would take into account the blood glucose chronodesm if the research hypothesis was not accepted. The platform was implemented in Java using NetBeans and PowerAMC

For this study, we did not interfere in the adaptation of patients' insulin doses. We limited ourselves to the implementation of an IT solution to help patients better adapt their insulin doses to their blood glucose levels.

- **NetBeans IDE**

NetBeans is an integrated development environment: a development tool that lets you write source code in Java and other languages such as Python, C, C++, JavaScript, XML, Ruby, PHP and HTML. Java is an object-oriented programming language, and one of its advantages is its portability .[35]

---

[34] ml: mean of sample1; m2: mean of sample 2; s1: variance of sample 1; s2: variance of sample 2

[35] Any program coded in Java must be usable with all operating systems on which a Java virtual machine is installed. In fact, when the source code is compiled, it takes on an intermediate form called byte code,

Insulin dose adjustment was based on glycemic and glycosuric targets. Clearly, the ideal was to achieve :

- absence of sugars in urine
- blood sugar levels
    - between 70 and 100 mg/dl
    - postprandial < 160mg/dl.

The insulin dose adaptation algorithm is based on the following general rules proposed by H. Dorchy[36] :

- if the target is reached, the same dose of insulin is left on the next day to act at the same time as the glycemic or glycosuric measurement, unless you plan to modify your diet and/or physical activity.
- if there are signs of hypoglycemia and/or blood glucose < 70mg/dl, during the period of action of the insulin considered[37] , the following day this insulin is reduced by 10% (minimum ½ unit). This is on condition that the patient has not eaten less than usual or engaged in unplanned physical activity.
- if the blood glucose level is >160mg/dl during the period of action of the insulin in question, 2 or 3 days in a row at the same time of day, the dose is

---

which can be interpreted by the Java virtual machine. This is commonly referred to as the JRE (Java Runtime Environment).

[36] H. Dorchy, Choix des insulines et adaptation des doses, op. cit. , p. 23.

[37] Action period of rapid-acting insulins or **Type I**: (onset of action: 10 min to ½ h after injection, peak 1h30 to 3h; end: 6 to 8h); action period of intermediate-acting insulins or **Type II**: (onset of action: 1 to 2 h after injection, peak 6h to 14h; end: 18 to 24h); action period of long-acting insulins or **Type III**: (onset of action: 3 to 4 h after injection, delayed action; end: 24 to 28h)

increased by 10% (minimum ½ unit) the following day, provided the patient has not eaten more than usual or had less physical activity.

Dose adjustment is therefore based primarily on retrospective examination of the previous days' results, and not solely on analysis of the moment immediately preceding the insulin injection.

- **PowerAMC,**

PowerDesigner is a software package that can be used to create all types of computer models. We used it to design the insulin dose adaptation algorithm (fig.5).

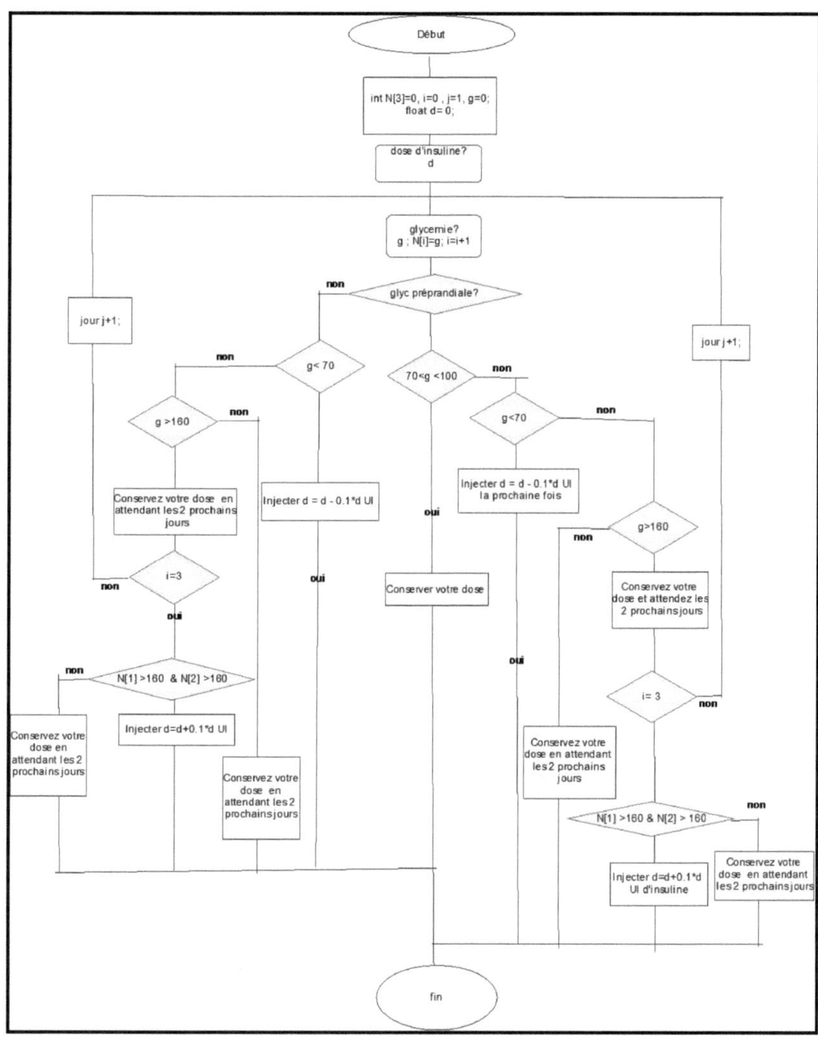

Figure 5 Insulin dose adaptation algorithm

IV. RESULTS AND DISCUSSIONS

1. OVERALL AND DESCRIPTIVE RESULTS

Over the study period, 9 patients (2 males and 7 females) were included: a sex ratio (males/females) of 0.28. The mean age was 27.2 years (extremes 13 and 44 years). All were type 1 diabetics. The average length of their diabetes was 13.1 years (extremes 1 and 23 years). Table 1 shows the profile of patients according to age and length of diabetes.

SUBJECT	AGE (years)	YEARS OF DIABETES (years)
Patient 1	24	17
Patient 2	26	13
Patient 3	34	23
Patient 4	23	19
Patient 5	20	9
Patient 6	36	12
Patient 7	25	1
Patient 8	13	1
Patient 9	44	23

Table 1Distribution of patients by age and length of diabetes

During conventional control, the average time at which patients usually checked their blood glucose levels was 08h01min. Table 2 shows the average profile of patients' hourly blood glucose monitoring habits.

SUBJECT	AVERAGE TIME OF GLYCEMIA INTAKE (h, min)
Patient 1	9 :34
Patient 2	07 :48
Patient 3	07 :41
Patient 4	07 :20
Patient 5	08 :36
Patient 6	09 :38
Patient 7	08 :16
Patient 8	07 :59
Patient 9	05 :19

Table 2Patients' usual average glycemic control schedule

Mean blood glucose levels were 1.71 g/l for conventional control and 1.72 g/l for chronobiological control. The mean HbA1c level was 8.7% for the conventional control and 9% for the chronobiological control. Figures 6 to 14 show the blood glucose profiles between the conventional and chronobiological controls in the various patients in our study. In no patient was blood glucose stable over the month, whatever the type of control. Chronobiological control did not appear to be any more effective than conventional control in improving patients' glycemic control.

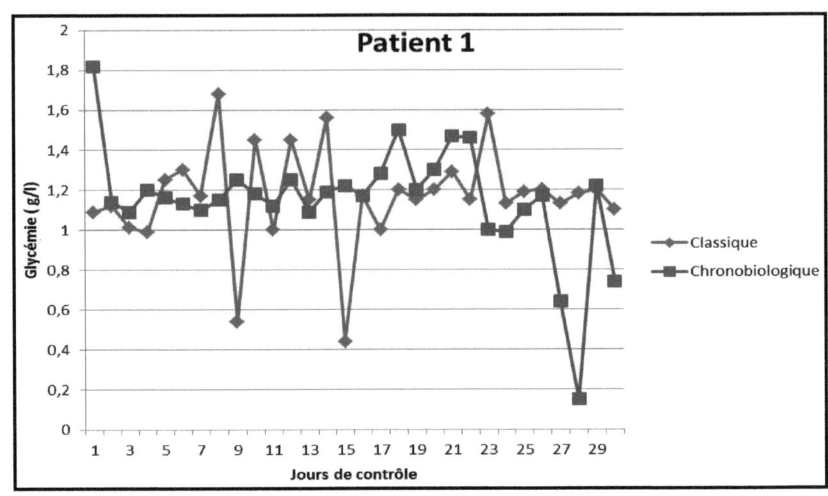

Figure 6 Glycemic profile of patient 1 during two types of follow-up

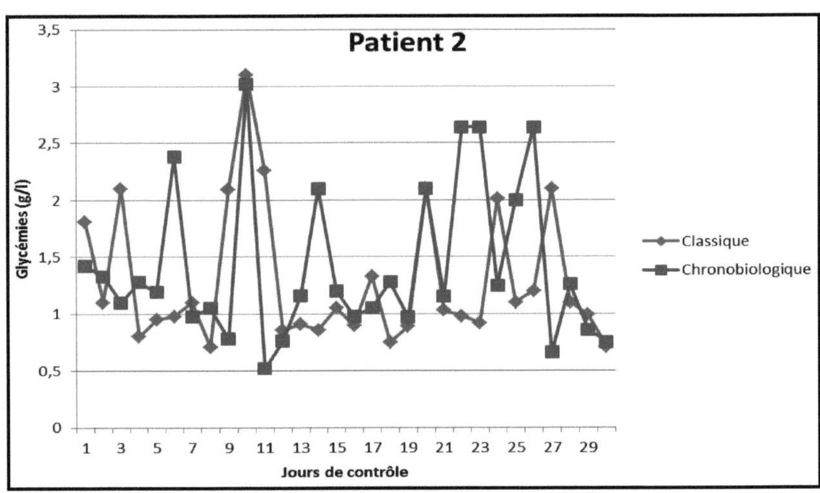

Figure 7 Glycemic profile of patient 2 for both types of follow-up

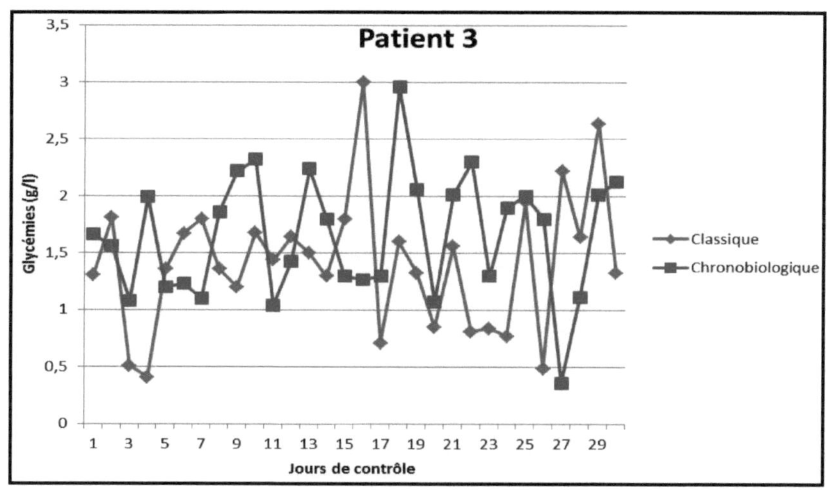

Figure 8 Glycemic profile of patient 3 during both follow-up procedures

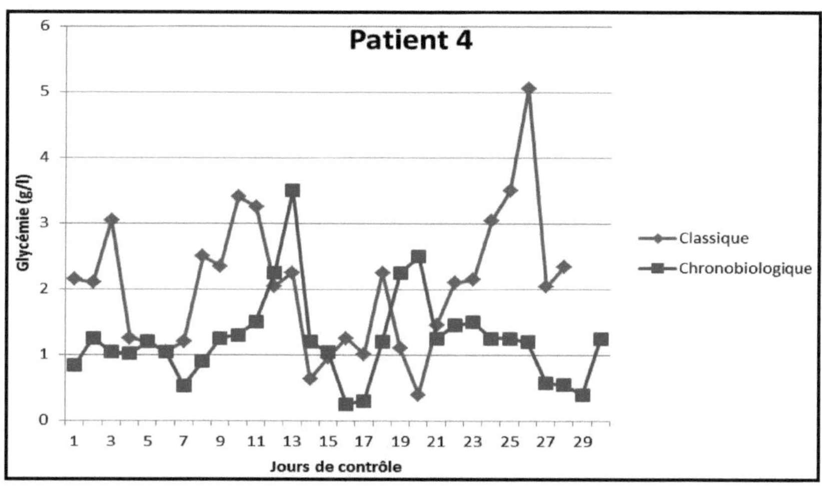

Figure 9 Patient 4's glycemic profile for both types of follow-up

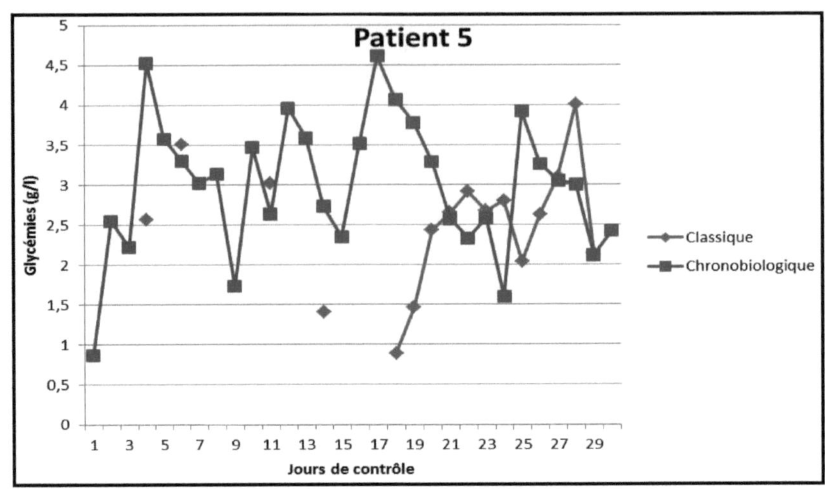

<u>Figure 10</u>Glycemic profile of patient 5 for both follow-up procedures

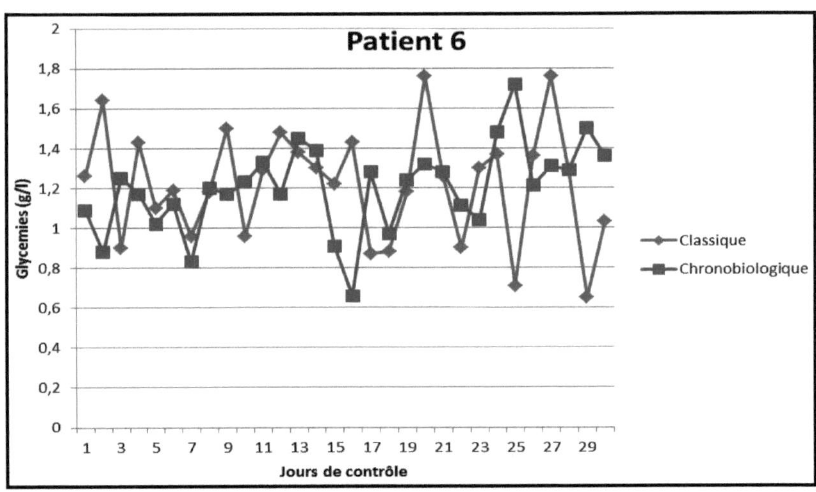

<u>Figure 11</u>Glycemic profile of patient 6 for both types of follow-up

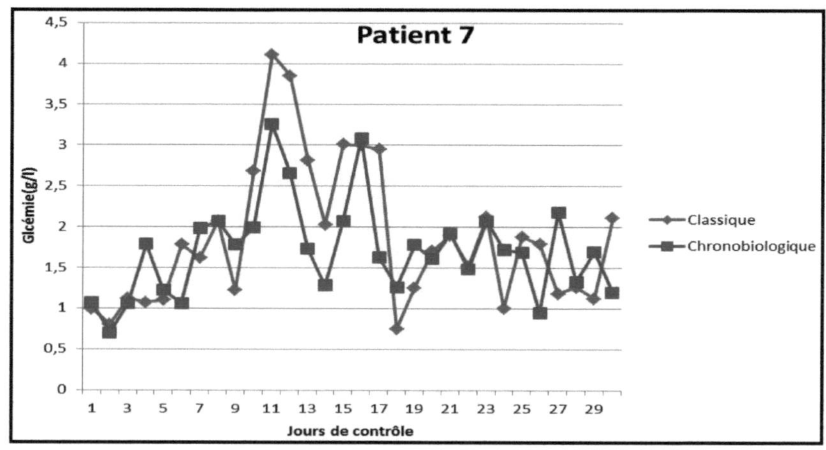

Figure 12Glycemic profile of patient 7 for the two types of follow-up

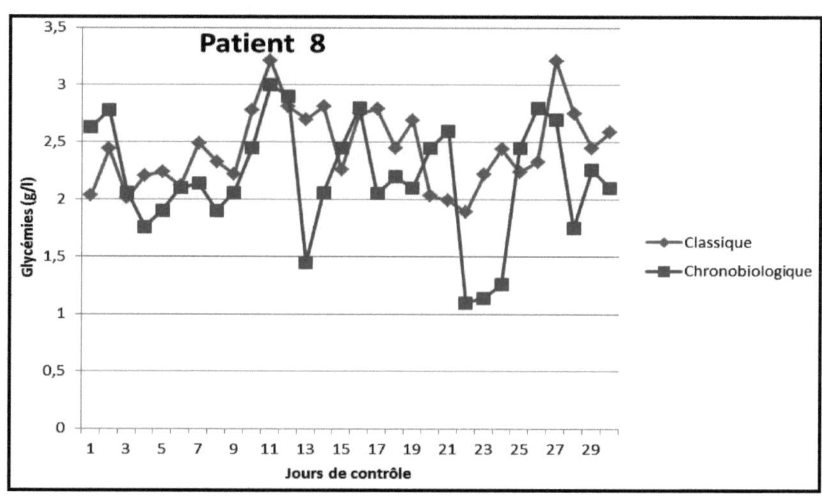

Figure 13Glycemic profile of patient 8 for both types of follow-up

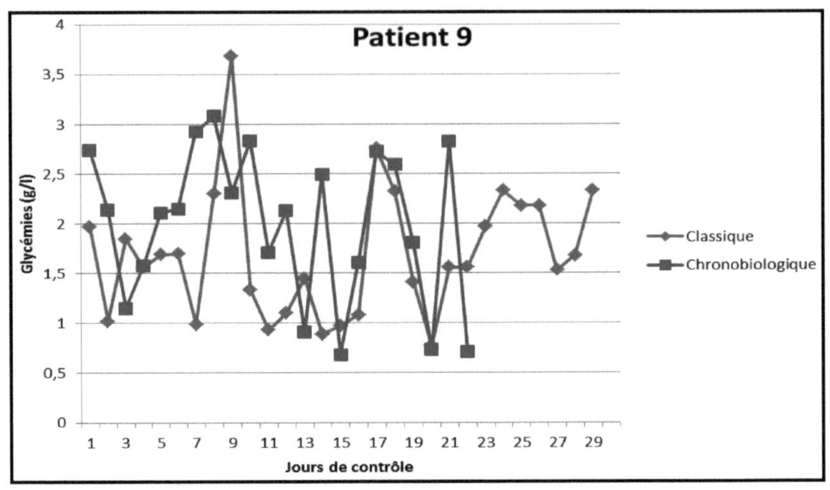

Figure 14Glycemic profile of patient 9 for both types of monitoring

The overall visualization of patient results was represented by the histograms in figures 15 and 16. These histograms showed the differences between mean blood glucose levels and HbA1c values observed in patients during the two types of follow-up. Patients 1, 4, 5, 6 and 7 showed lower mean blood glucose levels in chronobiological control. Patients 2; 3; 7 and 9 showed a drop in glycated hemoglobin in chronobiological control. In all, 5 out of 9 patients experienced a fall in their average blood glucose level: a percentage of 55%. In the case of HbA1c, only 4 out of 9 patients had a lower result: a percentage of 44%.

Histograms of HbA1c levels according to patient age (fig.17) and length of diabetes (fig.18) showed a link between glycemic control and both patient age and length of diabetes. Indeed, the older the patient, the better his glycemic control, although chronobiological control was not found to be superior (fig.17). The same observation was made in relation to the age of diabetes (fig.18). The longer the diabetes, the better the patient's glycemic control. However, chronobiological control was not superior to conventional control.

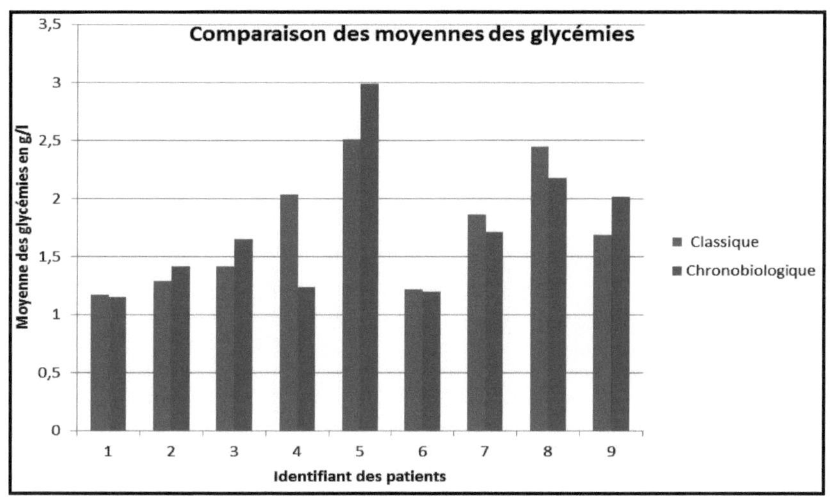

Figure 15 Histograms comparing blood glucose averages

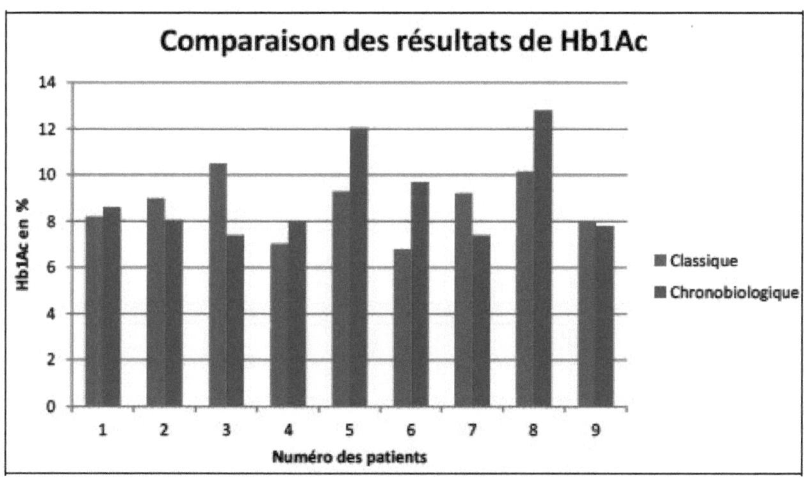

Figure 16 Histograms comparing dHbA1c levels

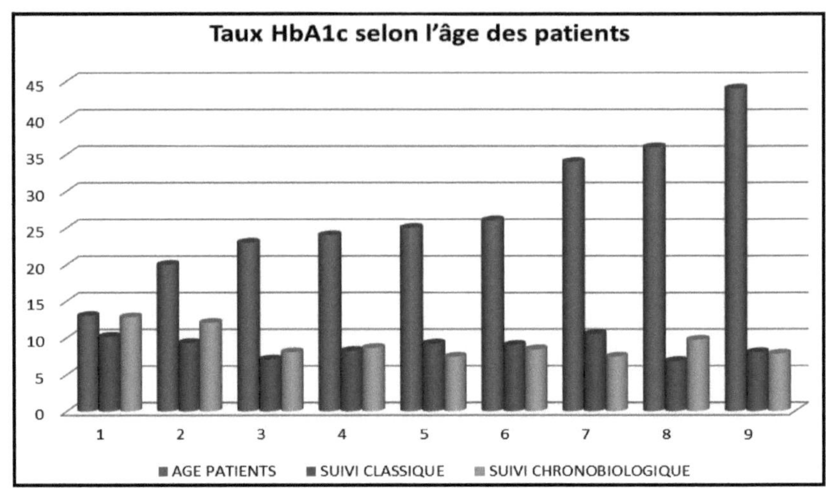

Figure 17 Histograms comparing HbA1c levels by patient age

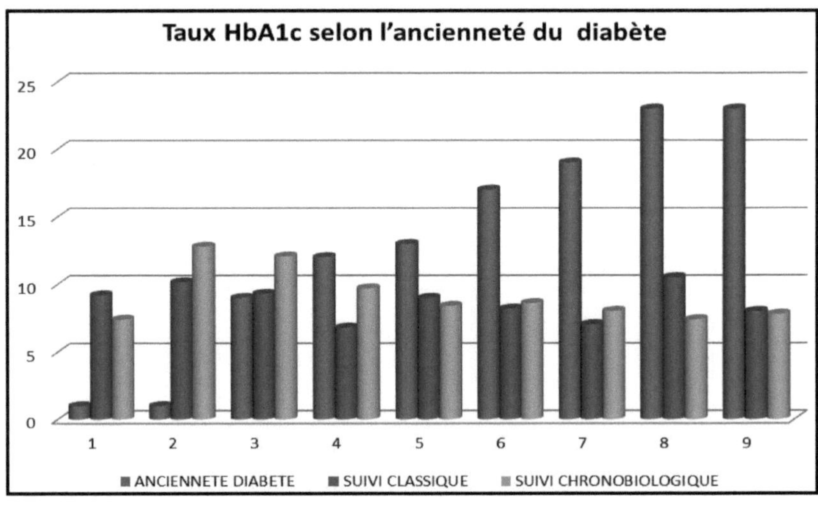

Figure 18 Histograms comparing HbA1c levels by age of diabetes

Comparison with the whisker boxes (figs. 19 and 20) already suggested an 'intuitive' reading of the differences. Figure 19 showed 3 atypical values for the classical control and 4 for the chronobiological control. We also noticed that the medians of each control were not centered in their boxes, and the whiskers are asymmetrical. The distribution of the two samples did not appear to be normal (non-centered medians, symmetry) and the approximate equality of variances did not appear to have been achieved (interquartile ranges were not of the same size). The median of the classical control was slightly higher than that of the chronobiological control; the two boxes overlapped a little, which tended to indicate a less significant difference between these two types of control.

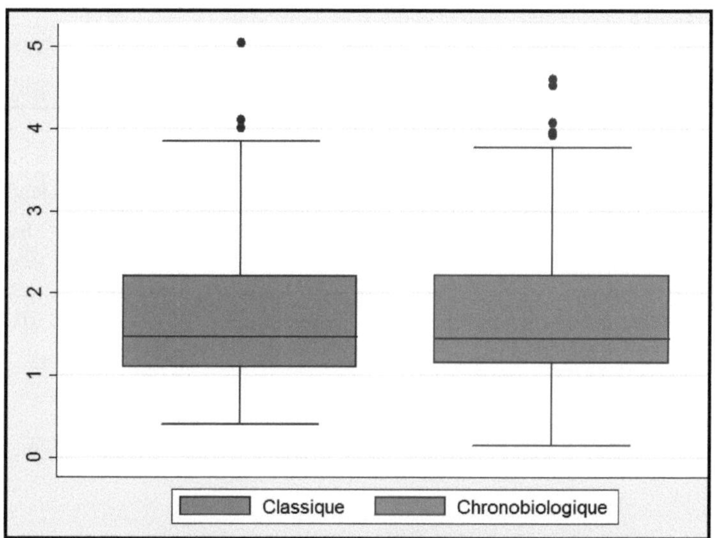

Figure 19Comparison of glycemia variable by type of follow-up

The same type of comparison could be made with HbA1c levels in figure 20. It was noticeable that the distribution did not appear to be normal, and that equality of variance was far from being achieved. A single atypical point was observed for chronobiological control. The two boxes overlapped slightly, and the median of the classical control was higher than that of the chronobiological control.

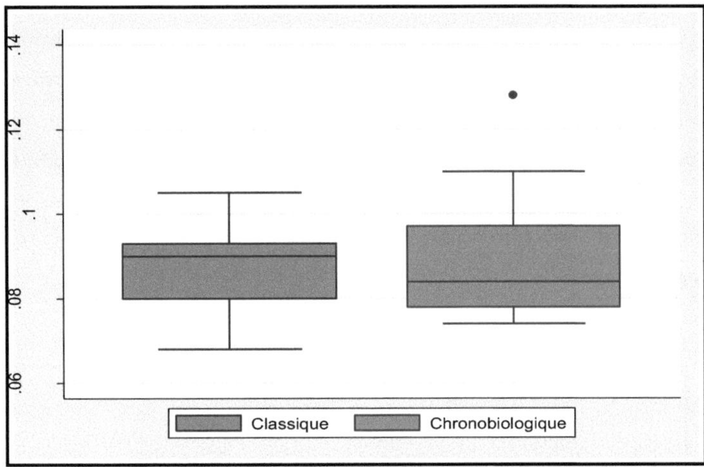

Figure 20Comparison of HbA1c levels by type of follow-up

This visual comparison probably needed to be confirmed by Student's mean comparison test. The conditions for applying the mean comparison test[38] had to be checked beforehand.

Under the null hypothesis of normality, the Shapiro-Wilks test (figs. 10 and 11) was used to calculate the statistics for the blood glucose and HbA1c variables:

- For blood glucose

[38] Conditions for applying the comparison of means test :

- Test samples must be taken at random;
- samples must follow a normal distribution: normality ;
- samples must have homogeneous variances: homoscedasticity.

H_0 : The **classic** distribution is normal (respectively the **chronobiological** distribution is normal).

H_1 : The **classical** distribution is not normal (respectively the **chronobiological** distribution is not normal).

Variable	Obs	W	V	z	Prob>z
	Shapiro-Wilk W test for normal data				
classique	254	0.93476	11.998	5.786	0.00000
chronobiol~e	263	0.93476	12.372	5.867	0.00000

Figure 21Screenshot of blood glucose normality test

p-value[39] $_{classic}$<5% ; p-value $_{chronobiological}$<5% . We reject H_0 : these two variables are therefore not normal.

- For HbA1c levels

The same assumptions apply.

```
. swilk classique chronobiologique
```

Variable	Obs	W	V	z	Prob>z
	Shapiro-Wilk W test for normal data				
classique	9	0.95798	0.617	-0.762	0.77698
chronobiol~e	9	0.84703	2.247	1.482	0.06911

Figure 22Screenshot of HbA1c normality test

$_{classic}$ p-value >5%; $_{chronobiological}$ p-value >5%. We accept H_0 : these two variables are therefore normal.

As the blood glucose distribution is not Gaussian, the Wilcoxon test will be used to compare means. Only the homoscedasticity of the variable HbA1c is verified. Under

[39] The p-values are calculated in the Prob>z column.

the null hypothesis of equality of variances of the variables (fig. 23), the statistic is calculated using Levene's test .[40]

p-value[41] $_{classic}$ >5% ; p-value $_{chronobiological}$ >5% . We accept H_0 : the variance of these two controls is of the same magnitude.

- For HbA1c levels

$H_0 : s'_1 = s'_2$; $H_1 : s'_1 \neq s'_2$

Variance ratio test

Variable	Obs	Mean	Std. Err.	Std. Dev.	[95% Conf.	Interval]
classi~e	9	.0867222	.0041991	.0125974	.077039	.0964054
chrono~e	9	.0901333	.0061202	.0183606	.0760202	.1042465
combined	18	.0884278	.003624	.0153753	.0807818	.0960737

```
    ratio = sd(classique) / sd(chronobiologique)                    f =   0.4707
Ho: ratio = 1                                      degrees of freedom =     8, 8

    Ha: ratio < 1               Ha: ratio != 1                 Ha: ratio > 1
  Pr(F < f) = 0.1535         2*Pr(F < f) = 0.3071           Pr(F > f) = 0.8465
```

Figure 23Screenshot of HbA1c equality of variance test

$_{classic}$ p-value >5%; $_{chronobiological}$ p-value >5%. We accept H_0 : the variance of these two controls is of the same magnitude.

Since both conditions - normality and homoscedasticity - are satisfied for HbA1c, we can easily apply *Student's t-test* for comparison of means. Assuming the null hypothesis of equality of means, we calculate the Wilcoxon statistic for blood glucose and the Student statistic for HbA1c (fig. 24 and 25).

---

[40] This test is less sensitive to distortion of the normal distribution (observed in the case of blood glucose) than Fisher's and Bartlett's tests.

[41] The p-value is calculated at the bottom of the table: 2*Pr (F < f)

- For blood glucose

$H_0 : m_1 = m_2$; $H_1 : m_1 > m_2$

```
Sign test

        sign |    observed    expected
-------------+------------------------
    positive |         123         121
    negative |         119         121
        zero |           5           5
-------------+------------------------
         all |         247         247

One-sided tests:
  Ho: median of classique - chronobiologique = 0 vs.
  Ha: median of classique - chronobiologique > 0
      Pr(#positive >= 123) =
         Binomial(n = 242, x >= 123, p = 0.5) =  0.4236

  Ho: median of classique - chronobiologique = 0 vs.
  Ha: median of classique - chronobiologique < 0
      Pr(#negative >= 119) =
         Binomial(n = 242, x >= 119, p = 0.5) =  0.6260

Two-sided test:
  Ho: median of classique - chronobiologique = 0 vs.
  Ha: median of classique - chronobiologique != 0
      Pr(#positive >= 123 or #negative >= 123) =
         min(1, 2*Binomial(n = 242, x >= 123, p = 0.5)) =  0.8471
```

Figure 24Screenshot of Wilcoxon blood glucose test

p-value[42] $_{classic}$ >5%; p-value $_{chronobiological}$ >5%. We accept H_0 : there was no significant difference between the blood glucose values obtained during the two types of control.

42 The p-value is calculated at the bottom of the table: Pr (#positive >= 126 or # negative >=126)

- For HbA1c levels

$H_0 : m'_1 = m'_2$; $H_1 : m'_1 > m'_2$

```
. ttest classique==chronobiologique

Paired t test
------------------------------------------------------------------------------
Variable |     Obs        Mean    Std. Err.   Std. Dev.   [95% Conf. Interval]
---------+--------------------------------------------------------------------
classi~e |       9    .0867222    .0041991    .0125974     .077039    .0964054
chrono~e |       9    .0901333    .0061202    .0183606    .0760202    .1042465
---------+--------------------------------------------------------------------
    diff |       9   -.0034111    .0067127    .0201382   -.0188907    .0120685
------------------------------------------------------------------------------
     mean(diff) = mean(classique - chronobiologique)              t =  -0.5082
 Ho: mean(diff) = 0                              degrees of freedom =        8

 Ha: mean(diff) < 0           Ha: mean(diff) != 0           Ha: mean(diff) > 0
 Pr(T < t) = 0.3125         Pr(|T| > |t|) = 0.6251          Pr(T > t) = 0.6875
```

Figure 25 Screenshot of Student's t test of HbA1c levels

p-value $_{classic}$ >5% ; p-value $_{chronobiological}$ >5% . We accept H_0 : there was no significant difference between the HbA1c levels obtained during the two types of control.

As the test was not significant, the parameters of our application did not take into account the blood glucose chronodesm. In order to verify the functionality of our software solution, we carried out a test using fasting blood glucose data from three (3) randomly selected patients on the first three days of chronobiological control (Tab. 2). By repnding 'true' to the question "Is this a preprandial blood glucose level? you inform the application that you have fasting blood glucose and 'false', the opposite case.

	Patient1		Patient4		Patient8	
Days	Blood glucose (g/l)	Insulin dose	Blood glucose (g/l)	Insulin dose	Blood glucose (g/l)	Insulin dose
1	1,82	12-12 Mixt	0,84	10-10-10 Act / 0-8-0 Mixt	2,63	12-12-12 Act
2	1,14	12-12 Mixt	1,25	12-12-12 Act / 0-8-0 Mixt	2,78	12-12-12 Act

3	1,09	12-12 Mixt	1,04	14-14-14 Act / 0-8-0 Mixt	2,06	12-12-12 Act

Table 3Actual data for patients 1, 4, 8 during the first three days of chronobiological monitoring

For patient 1, our application proposed that his insulin dose be maintained after monitoring his data for three (3) consecutive days (fig.27). Although the same proposal was made to patient 4, it should be noted that the treatment did not require data from the following two (2) days, as his blood glucose levels were normal (fig.28). Similarly, the application would have suggested that he switch to a morning dose of 9 IU Mixtard (i.e. reduce his insulin dose by 10%) if his blood glucose was below 70 mg/dl. As for patient 8, after monitoring his data over three (3) consecutive days, the application suggested (fig.29) that he switch to a morning dose of 13.2 IU of Actrapid (i.e. increase his insulin dose by 10%).

```
run:
---Adaptation de la dose d'insuline chez les diabétiques de type 1---
Entrez votre dose d'insuline
12
Entrez votre glycémie durant le temps d'action de l'insuline
182
Est-ce une glycémie préprandiale? true/false
true
Hyperglycémie: conservez votre dose d'insuline et atttendez les 2 prochains jours
---Jour 2---
 Entrez votre glycémie durant le temps d'action de l'insuline du jour  2
114
Est-ce une glycemie preprandiale? true/false
true
Glycémie légèrement au dessus de la normale: Conserver votre dose
---Jour 3---
 Entrez votre glycémie durant le temps d'action de l'insuline du jour  3
109
Est-ce une glycemie preprandiale? true/false
true
Glycémie légèrement au dessus de la normale: Conserver votre dose
Bilan des 3 jours:conservez votre dose d'insuline et atttendez les 2 prochains jours
BUILD SUCCESSFUL (total time: 57 seconds)
```

Figure 26 Screenshot of insulin adaptation proposal for patient 1

```
run:
---Adaptation de la dose d'insuline chez les diabétiques de type 1---
Entrez votre dose d'insuline
10
Entrez votre glycémie durant le temps d'action de l'insuline
84
Est-ce une glycémie préprandiale? true/false
true
Glycémie normale: conservez votre dose d'insuline
BUILD SUCCESSFUL (total time: 46 seconds)
```

Figure 27 Screenshot of patient 4's insulin proposal

```
run:
---Adaptation de la dose d'insuline chez les diabétiques de type 1---
Entrez votre dose d'insuline
12
Entrez votre glycémie durant le temps d'action de l'insuline
263
Est-ce une glycémie préprandiale? true/false
true
Hyperglycémie: conservez votre dose d'insuline et atttendez les 2 prochains jours
---Jour 2---
 Entrez votre glycémie durant le temps d'action de l'insuline du jour  2
278
Est-ce une glycemie preprandiale? true/false
true
Hyperglycémie: conservez votre dose d'insuline et atttendez le prochain jour
---Jour 3---
 Entrez votre glycémie durant le temps d'action de l'insuline du jour  3
206
Est-ce une glycemie preprandiale? true/false
true

Injectez 13.2 UI d'insuline la prochaine fois
BUILD SUCCESSFUL (total time: 50 seconds)
```

Figure 28 Screenshot of patient 8's insulin adaptation proposal

Table 4 Summary of blood glucose and glycated hemoglobin values for each patient, by type of control

Patient (p)	Control type	Classic (c1)										Chronobiological (c2)									
1	Blood glucose	1,0	1,1	1,0	0,9	1,2	1,3	1,1	1,6	0,5	1,4	1,8	1,1	1,0	1,2	1,1	1,1	1,1	1,1	1,2	1,1
		1	1,4	1,1	1,5	0,4	1,1	1	1,2	1,1	1,2	1,1	1,2	1,0	1,1	1,2	1,1	1,2	1,5	1,2	1,3
		1,2	1,1	1,5	1,1	1,1	1,2	1,1	1,1	1,2	1,1	1,4	1,4	1	0,9	1,1	1,1	0,6	0,1	1,2	0,7
	HbA1c(	8,2										8,6									
2	Blood glucose	1,8	1,1	2,1	0,8	0,9	0,9	1,1	0,7	2,0	3,1	1,8	1,1	2,1	0,8	0,9	0,9	1,1	0,7	2,0	3,1
		2,2	0,8	0,9	0,8	1,0	0,9	1,3	0,7	0,8	2,1	2,2	0,8	0,9	0,8	1,0	0,9	1,3	0,7	0,8	2,1
		1,0	0,9	0,9	2,0	1,1	1,2	2,1	1,1	0,9	0,7	1,0	0,9	0,9	2,0	1,1	1,2	2,1	1,1	0,9	0,7
	HbA1c(	9										8,4									
3	Blood glucose	1,3	1,8	0,5	0,4	1,3	1,6	1,8	1,3	1,2	1,6	1,6	1,5	1,0	1,9	1,2	1,2	1,1	1,8	2,2	2,3
		1,4	1,6	1,5	1,3	1,8	3	0,7	1,6	1,3	0,8	1,0	1,4	2,2	1,8	1,3	1,2	1,3	2,9	2,0	1,0
		1,5	0,8	0,8	0,7	1,9	0,4	2,2	1,6	2,6	1,3	2,0	2,3	1,3	1,9	2	1,8	0,3	1,1	2,0	2,1
	HbA1c(%)	10,5										7,4									

		Classic										Chronobiological									
4	Blood glucose	2,1	2,1	3,0	1,2	1,2	1,0	1,2	2,5	2,3	3,4	0,8	1,2	1,0	1,0	1,2	1,0	0,5	0,9	1,2	1,3
		3,2	2,0	2,2	0,6	0,9	1,2	1,0	2,2	1,1	0,4	1,5	2,2	3,5	1,2	1,0	0,2	0,3	1,2	2,2	2,5
		1,4	2,1	2,1	3,0	3,5	5,0	2,0	2,3	NA	NA	1,2	1,4	1,5	1,2	1,2	1,2	0,5	0,5	0,4	1,2
	HbA1c(	7,05										8,02									
5	Blood glucose	NA	NA	NA	2,5	2,5	3,5	NA	NA	NA	NA	0,8	2,5	2,2	4,5	3,5	3,3	3,0	3,1	1,7	3,4
		3,0	NA	NA	1,4	NA	NA	NA	0,8	1,4	2,4	2,6	3,9	3,5	2,7	2,3	3,5	4,6	4,0	3,7	3,2
		2,6	2,9	2,6	2,8	2,0	2,6	3,1	4,0	2,1	NA	2,5	2,3	2,5	1,6	3,9	3,2	3,0	3	2,1	2,4
	HbA1c(	9,3										12,05									
6	Blood glucose	1,2	1,6	0,9	1,4	1,1	1,1	0,9	1,1	1,5	0,9	1,0	0,8	1,2	1,1	1,0	1,1	0,8	1,2	1,1	1,2
		1,2	1,4	1,3	1,3	1,2	1,4	0,8	0,8	1,1	1,7	1,3	1,1	1,4	1,3	0,9	0,6	1,2	0,9	1,2	1,3
		1,2	0,9	1,3	1,3	0,7	1,3	1,7	1,2	0,6	1,0	1,2	1,1	1,0	1,4	1,7	1,2	1,3	1,2	1,5	1,3
	HbA1c(	6,8										9,7									
7	Blood glucos	0,9	0,8	1,1	1,0	1,1	1,7	1,6	2,0	1,2	2,6	1,0	0,7	1,0	1,7	1,2	1,0	1,9	2,0	1,7	1,9
		4,1	3,8	2,8	2,0	3,0	3	2,9	0,7	1,2	1,7	3,2	2,6	1,7	1,2	2,0	3,0	1,6	1,2	1,7	1,6

		1,9	1,5	2,1	1	1,8	1,7	1,1	1,2	1,1	2,1	1,9	1,4	2,0	1,7	1,6	0,9	2,1	1,3	1,7	1,2
	HbA1c(	9,2										7,4									

		Classic										Chronobiological									
8	Blood glucose	2,0	2,4	2,0	2,2	2,2	2,1	2,4	2,3	2,2	2,7	2,6	2,7	2,0	1,7	1,9	2,1	2,1	1,9	2,0	2,4
		3,2	2,8	2,7	2,8	2,2	2,7	2,7	2,4	2,6	2,0	3	2,9	1,4	2,0	2,4	2,8	2,0	2,2	2,1	2,4
		1,9	1,8	2,2	2,4	2,2	2,3	3,2	2,7	2,4	2,5	2,6	1,1	1,1	1,2	2,4	2,8	2,7	1,7	2,2	2,1
	HbA1c(%)	10										12,8									
9	Blood glucose	1,5	1,9	1,0	1,8	1,5	1,6	1,7	0,9	2,3	3,6	2,3	2,7	2,1	1,1	1,5	2,1	2,1	2,9	3,0	2,3
		1,3	0,9	1,1	1,4	0,8	0,9	1,0	2,7	2,3	1,4	2,8	1,7	2,1	0,9	2,4	0,6	1,6	2,7	2,5	1,8
		0,7	1,5	1,5	1,9	2,3	2,1	2,1	1,5	1,6	2,3	0,7	2,8	0,7	NA	NA	NA	NA	NA	NA	NA
	HbA1c(%)	8										7,8									

2. INTERPRETATION

Tests comparing blood glucose and HbA1c levels for the two types of control confirmed the null hypothesis of equality of means. The observed differences in mean blood glucose and HbA1c levels were therefore not significant enough to confirm the efficacy of chronobiological control compared with conventional control. Thus, fasting blood glucose control according to the biological clock had no significant effect on glycemic control in type 1 diabetics, and hence on insulin dose adjustment. Thus, the parameters of the insulin dose adaptation agorithm did not take into account the biological clock.

3. DISCUSSIONS

Managing diabetics requires self-monitoring to ensure optimum glycemic control.

We tested the hypothesis that there was no significant difference between fasting capillary blood glucose levels obtained at any time of the morning and those obtained at the acrophase of the blood glucose cycle. The aim was to test the hypothesis that control according to the biological clock provides type 1 diabetics with an additional benefit in terms of self-monitoring of their blood glucose levels, with implications for the insulin dose they need to inject.

Type 1 diabetes manifests itself at a young age. This explains why the average age of our study population was 27.2 years. This type of diabetes was called juvenile diabetes by the WHO. The 'right' treatment for type 1 diabetes is one that achieves an HbA1c level below 7% without severe hypoglycemia. However, the average blood glucose and HbA1c levels obtained in our study (8.7% for conventional control and 9% for chronobiological control) fall far short of the target. Indeed, chronobiological analysis of insulin sensitivity in type 1 diabetics revealed a magnitude[43] of 20% on average. This ratio, reflecting insulin resistance, is all the higher the less balanced the subjects (high HbA1c) . [44]

The different blood glucose and HbA1c results (1.71 g/l and 8.7% for conventional control versus 1.72 g/l and 9% for chronobiological control) obtained in this study did not allow us to invalidate the research hypothesis without risk of error. However, chronobiology tells us that biological rhythms can differ from one individual to another. This explains the drop in average blood glucose levels in 55% of patients and in HbA1c levels in 44% of patients.

It should be pointed out that our study suffered from a number of shortcomings, such as the small size of our sample, which is not representative of the type 1 diabetic population. In fact, type 1 diabetics represent around 10% of the 400,000 diabetics in Senegal[45] : a population of 40,000. This type of study requires us to supply the necessary glycometer strips to patients and to pay for their HbA1c assays. However, the financial means at our disposal were insufficient to envisage a representative sample of over 2,000 patients .[46]

We also had to contend with a number of biases, such as the one-month time interval between HbA1c determinations for each type of control. HbA1c levels reflect the patient's glycemic control over a 3-month period. For better interpretation of glycemic control as reflected by the HbA1c level, it was necessary to extend the study duration from sixty (60) days to two hundred and forty (240) days. The constraints created by

---

[43] Percentage increase in insulin requirements at the end of the night versus the beginning of the night

[44] Eric Marsaudon, Chronobiologie et diabète. op. cit. , p. 14.

[45] Dakar Actu, (21 /12/13). Diabetes in Senegal, *Cyberpresse*, [online], www.dakaractu.com, accessed 05/26/14.

[46] The required sample size is estimated at 2266 for an estimated response rate of 20%, a confidence interval of 95% and a margin of error of 2%.

changes in the chronobiological control habits of certain patients, as well as errors linked to incorrect meter handling, should not be ignored.

For future studies of similar comparison, it would be important to take a larger sample size, to put patients in the right conditions of care, and to extend the study over six(6) months for each patient. The insulin dose adaptation algorithm could be optimized to cover insulin intakes throughout the day, and take account of insulin combinations. This ap

V. CONCLUSION AND OUTLOOK

In the management of diabetic patients, chronobiology suggests that healthcare staff take time into account when measuring biological parameters that fluctuate on a nycthemeral basis, such as blood glucose, cortisol and cholesterol levels.

The results of our study failed to confirm the significant efficacy of chronobiology on glycemic control in type 1 diabetics. This is mainly due to the fact that we were unable to obtain a sufficiently representative sample of data on which to apply our statistical tests. Nevertheless, chronobiology's dynamic approach to the analysis of human physiology remains one of the major avenues open to tomorrow's medicine.

When it comes to self-monitoring of blood glucose levels, further large-scale comparative studies are needed, so that the WHO can incorporate physiological blood glucose variables (instead of biological constants) into its reference values. This would enable diabetic patients to compare their blood glucose levels, at any time of day, with references that take into account fluctuations in blood glucose levels.

BIBLIOGRAPHICAL REFERENCES

1. Association française des diabétiques, [online], www.afd.fr/Vivreaveclediabète/ Self-monitoring/, accessed on 01/23/14.

2. World Atlas 2003, page 8/58.

3. Bolli G.B., Circadian rhythms of insulin sensitivity and its role in the treatment of diabetes mellitus. In Biological cloks. Mechanisms and applications. Amsterdam Elsevier Science 1998: 405-409.

4. Bourdon L, Buguet A, Cucherat M, Radomski MW. Use of a spreadsheet program for circadian analysis of biological/physiological data. Aviat Space Environ Med, 1995; 66: 787-91.

5. Dakar Actu, (21 /12/13). Diabetes in Senegal, *Cyberpresse*, [online], www.dakaractu.com, accessed 05/26/14.

6. Eric Marsaudon, Chronobiologie et diabète. Rev La semaine des Hôpitaux de Paris, 1998; 74: 1148-1154.

7. Eric Marsaudon, La chronobiologie, une conception dynamique du fonctionnement corporel, Presses de Sciences Po | Les Tribunes de la santé 2006/4 - no 13 ; 39-44 ISSN 1765-8888.

8. International Diabetes Federation, Global Diabetes Plan 2011-2021, [online], www.idf.org/sites/default/files/attachments/GDP_FR.pdf, accessed 12/02/14.

9. Foley JP, Dorsey JG. A review of the exponentially modified gaussian (EMG) function: evaluation and subsequent calculation of universal data. J Chromatogr Sci 1984; 22: 40-6.

10. H. Dorchy, Choix des insulines et adaptation des doses chez les enfants et les adolescents diabétiques : expérience personnelle, *Rev Méd Brux 2000* ; 1 :19-27

11. Halberg, Franz. Solving some chronobiological puzzles of general application. *Bulletin du groupe d'étude des rythmes biologiques*, 1989 ; 1 : 36 -52.

12. Jean Michel Crabbé, De la biologie à la chronobiologie, [online], www.sitemed.fr, consulted on 30/08/12.

13. Jean-Michel Crabbé, Médecine et chronobiologie, I. les origines de la chronobiologie. L'échec de la médecine occidentale: l'idéologie médicale en question, Ellébore, 2003 :167-170.

14. Middeke M. Schrader J., Nocturmi blood pressure in normotensive subjects and those with white cont.primary and secondary hypertension, BMJ 1994; 308:630-632.

15. Nelson W, Tong YL, Lee J-K, Halberg F. Methods for cosinor rhythmometry. Chronobiologia, 1979;6:305-23.

16. Observatoire Africain de la Sante, lutte contre le Diabète sucre, [online], www.aho.afro.who.int/profiles_information/index.php/...Diabetes.../fr, accessed 12/02/14.

17. WHO Regional Office for Africa, Report of the Regional Director, Diabetes prevention and control: a strategy for the WHO African Region, 2007.

18. S. Halimi. Contributions of self-monitoring of blood glucose in the management of insulin-dependent (IDDM) and non-insulin-dependent (NIDDM) diabetics. *Diabetes & Metabolism* 1998, 24, 35-41.

19. Simon C. Brandenberger G., La pulsabilité de l'insulino-sécrétion, Rev Prat(Paris) 1994; 44, 6: 791-94

20. Sokolove PG, Bushell WN. The chi square periodogram: its utility for analysis of circadian rhythms. *J Theor Biol*, 1978; 8: 131-60.

21. Tattersall R. Homme glucose monitoring. *Diabetologia*, 1979, 16: 71-74.

TABLE OF CONTENTS

APPENDIX

Inquiry form

First and last name :

Tel:

Age :

Date	Time for blood glucose control	Blood glucose	Insulin dose

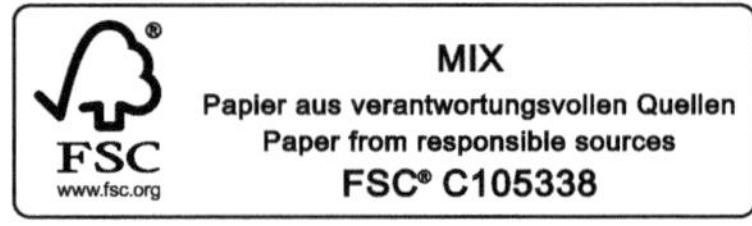

Printed by Books on Demand GmbH, Norderstedt / Germany